UNDERSTANDING DEMENTIA

Comprehensive Guide To Symptoms, Diagnosis, Treatment, And Care Strategies For Alzheimer's And Cognitive Decline

DR. LINCOLN WAYLON

Copyright © [2024] [Lincoln Waylon]. All Rights Reserved.

The copyright laws of the United States of America and other nations safeguard this publication. Except for brief quotations included in critical reviews and certain other non-commercial uses allowed by copyright law, no part of this book may be reproduced, distributed, or transmitted in any form or by any means, including photocopying, recording, or other electronic or mechanical methods, without the prior written permission of the copyright owner.

DISCLAIMER

This book contains information that should only be used for educational and informational reasons; it is not meant to be used as a source of medical or psychological advice. The author's studies, life experiences, and expertise in the area of health and wellness served as the foundation for the content. It should not, however, be used in place of expert counsel, a diagnosis, or medical care.

Any queries you may have about a physical or mental health issue should always be directed toward the advice of a licensed healthcare provider or mental health specialist. With regard to the efficacy or outcomes of the methods or suggestions included in this book, the author and publisher make no representations or warranties.

Any information or methods in this book are used entirely at the reader's own risk and discretion. The material provided here may be used or misused, and neither the author nor the publisher will be held responsible for any results, losses, or negative impacts.

Keep in mind that everyone has different demands and reactions to health and wellness routines. Any health and wellness plans you implement must be customized to your particular circumstances, and you should speak with experts to make sure the plans meet your needs.

TABLE OF CONTENTS

CHAPTER ONE 11
OVERVIEW OF DEMENTIA 11
- DEFINITION AND OVERVIEW 11
- DISTINCTION BETWEEN DEMENTIA AND NORMAL AGING 12
- TYPES OF DEMENTIA 14
- PREVALENCE AND IMPACT ON SOCIETY 15
- IMPORTANCE OF EARLY DIAGNOSIS AND INTERVENTION 17

CHAPTER TWO 19
DEMENTIA AND ITS IMPACT 19
- EFFECTS ON INDIVIDUALS AND FAMILIES 19
- EMOTIONAL AND PSYCHOLOGICAL IMPACT 20
- FINANCIAL AND SOCIAL IMPLICATIONS 22
- COPING WITH THE DIAGNOSIS 23
- SUPPORT SYSTEMS AND RESOURCES 25

CHAPTER THREE 27
BASICS OF BRAIN FUNCTION AND AGING 27
- HOW THE BRAIN FUNCTIONS NORMALLY 27
- CHANGES IN THE BRAIN WITH AGING 28
- HOW DEMENTIA AFFECTS BRAIN FUNCTION 30
- EARLY SIGNS AND SYMPTOMS 31
- DIAGNOSIS AND ASSESSMENT 33

CHAPTER FOUR 35
TYPES OF DEMENTIA 35
- ALZHEIMER'S DISEASE 35

- VASCULAR DEMENTIA 36
- LEWY BODY DEMENTIA 38
- FRONTOTEMPORAL DEMENTIA 39
- OTHER LESS COMMON TYPES 40

CHAPTER FIVE 43
- RISK FACTORS AND PREVENTION 43
  - GENETIC AND ENVIRONMENTAL RISK FACTORS 43
  - LIFESTYLE FACTORS AND PREVENTION STRATEGIES 44
  - ROLE OF DIET AND EXERCISE 46
  - COGNITIVE TRAINING AND MENTAL STIMULATION 47
  - IMPORTANCE OF REGULAR MEDICAL CHECK-UPS 48

CHAPTER SIX 49
- DIAGNOSIS AND TREATMENT 49
  - DIAGNOSTIC PROCESS AND TOOLS 49
  - MEDICAL AND COGNITIVE ASSESSMENTS 50
  - AVAILABLE TREATMENTS AND MEDICATIONS 52
  - ROLE OF CAREGIVERS AND FAMILY SUPPORT 53
  - ONGOING RESEARCH AND ADVANCEMENTS 55

CHAPTER SEVEN 57
- MANAGING DEMENTIA SYMPTOMS 57
  - BEHAVIORAL AND PSYCHOLOGICAL SYMPTOMS 57
  - TECHNIQUES FOR MANAGING CHALLENGING BEHAVIORS 59
  - STRATEGIES FOR IMPROVING QUALITY OF LIFE 60
  - IMPORTANCE OF ROUTINE AND STRUCTURE 62
  - ROLE OF OCCUPATIONAL THERAPY AND SUPPORT SERVICES 63

CHAPTER EIGHT 65
CAREGIVING AND SUPPORT 65
RESPONSIBILITIES OF CAREGIVERS 65
BALANCING CAREGIVING WITH PERSONAL LIFE 66
RESPITE CARE AND SUPPORT NETWORKS 68
LEGAL AND FINANCIAL CONSIDERATIONS 69
TRAINING AND RESOURCES FOR CAREGIVERS 71
CHAPTER NINE 73
LEGAL AND ETHICAL CONSIDERATIONS 73
LEGAL RIGHTS OF INDIVIDUALS WITH DEMENTIA 73
ADVANCE DIRECTIVES AND POWER OF ATTORNEY 74
ETHICAL DILEMMAS IN DEMENTIA CARE 76
GUARDIANSHIP AND DECISION-MAKING 77
PROTECTING PERSONAL AND FINANCIAL INTERESTS 78
CHAPTER TEN 81
FAQS 81
WHAT ARE THE COMMON SYMPTOMS OF DEMENTIA? 81
HOW IS DEMENTIA DIAGNOSED? 82
WHAT TREATMENTS ARE AVAILABLE FOR DEMENTIA? 84
HOW CAN CAREGIVERS TAKE CARE OF THEMSELVES? 85
WHAT IS THE ROLE OF RESEARCH IN DEMENTIA CARE? ... 87

ABOUT THE BOOK

"Understanding Dementia" provides a comprehensive and enlightening exploration of a condition that affects millions of individuals and their families worldwide. This book delves into the definition and overview of dementia, clarifying the distinction between dementia and normal aging, and exploring various types of dementia, including Alzheimer's disease, vascular dementia, Lewy body dementia, and frontotemporal dementia. By examining the prevalence and societal impact of these conditions, the book underscores the critical importance of early diagnosis and intervention in managing dementia.

The emotional, psychological, financial, and social implications of dementia are profoundly examined, highlighting the significant impact on both individuals and their families. The book provides invaluable insights into coping with a dementia diagnosis and navigating the associated challenges. It also offers guidance on leveraging support systems and resources to better manage the effects of dementia on daily life.

In understanding dementia, it is essential to grasp the basics of brain function and aging. The book elucidates how the brain functions under normal circumstances and what changes occur with aging. It further explains how dementia disrupts these processes, highlighting early signs and symptoms that can lead to a timely diagnosis. The diagnostic process is thoroughly covered, including medical and cognitive assessments, with a focus on available treatments and medications. The role of caregivers and family support in managing dementia is also discussed, along with ongoing research and advancements in the field.

Managing dementia symptoms is another critical area addressed, including techniques for handling behavioral and psychological challenges, strategies for improving quality of life, and the importance of routine and structure.

The book emphasizes the role of occupational therapy and support services in enhancing the lives of those affected by dementia.

Caregiving is a central theme, with detailed insights into the responsibilities of caregivers, balancing caregiving with personal life, and exploring respite care and support networks. Legal and financial considerations, including legal rights, advance directives, power of attorney, and ethical dilemmas in dementia care, are examined to guide caregivers and families in protecting personal and financial interests.

The book addresses frequently asked questions about dementia, providing clear answers on symptoms, diagnosis, treatments, caregiver self-care, and the role of research. "Understanding Dementia" stands as a vital resource, offering both depth and clarity in navigating the complexities of dementia care and support.

CHAPTER ONE
OVERVIEW OF DEMENTIA
DEFINITION AND OVERVIEW

Dementia is an umbrella term for a range of cognitive impairments that affect memory, thinking, and reasoning to the extent that daily functioning becomes difficult. It is characterized by a decline from a previously higher level of cognitive ability, impacting various aspects of a person's life, including their ability to perform everyday tasks and maintain relationships. This progressive condition results from damage to brain cells, which disrupts their ability to communicate effectively, leading to significant cognitive and behavioral changes.

The symptoms of dementia can vary depending on the type and severity of the disease. Common symptoms include memory loss, confusion, difficulty with language, and problems with reasoning and judgment.

As the condition advances, these symptoms can become more pronounced, leading to greater challenges in managing daily life. Understanding dementia involves recognizing these changes and knowing how they can affect individuals and their families over time.

To manage dementia effectively, it's crucial to identify the specific type of dementia early on, as treatment and support strategies can vary. Early recognition allows for timely intervention, which can help in managing symptoms and improving quality of life. Support from healthcare professionals, caregivers, and community resources play a vital role in providing comprehensive care and enhancing the overall well-being of those affected by dementia.

DISTINCTION BETWEEN DEMENTIA AND NORMAL AGING

While dementia and normal aging may share some similarities, such as memory lapses or slower cognitive processing, they are fundamentally different in their causes and impacts. Normal aging involves gradual changes in cognitive functions that typically do not interfere significantly with daily life. Memory problems experienced during aging are usually mild and do not worsen rapidly. For instance, occasional forgetfulness, like misplacing keys, is common and not necessarily indicative of a serious condition.

In contrast, dementia involves more severe and progressive cognitive decline that impacts daily functioning. This decline is not a normal part of aging but rather a result of specific neurological changes or diseases. Symptoms of dementia often include persistent memory loss, confusion, and difficulty with problem-solving that progressively interfere with the person's ability to live independently. Understanding this distinction helps in recognizing when memory and cognitive changes might warrant further evaluation and intervention.

The key to differentiating dementia from normal aging is to observe the progression and impact of symptoms.

Dementia symptoms tend to worsen over time and significantly impair daily activities, whereas age-related cognitive changes are generally stable and manageable. If memory problems or cognitive changes are persistent and interfere with daily life, seeking medical advice is important for proper diagnosis and treatment.

TYPES OF DEMENTIA

Dementia encompasses several types, each with distinct characteristics and underlying causes. Alzheimer's disease is the most common type, marked by gradual memory loss and confusion due to the buildup of amyloid plaques and tau tangles in the brain. Vascular dementia, another common type, arises from reduced blood flow to the brain, often following a stroke, and is characterized by difficulties with planning, reasoning, and memory.

Other types of dementia include Lewy body dementia, which involves abnormal protein deposits in brain cells and can cause fluctuations in alertness, visual hallucinations, and motor symptoms similar to Parkinson's disease. Frontotemporal dementia affects the frontal and temporal lobes of the brain, leading to changes in personality, behavior, and language. Understanding these different types of dementia helps in tailoring treatment and care approaches to the specific needs of individuals.

Each type of dementia requires a different management strategy and support system. Diagnosis typically involves a combination of medical history, cognitive tests, brain imaging, and sometimes genetic testing. Accurate identification of the type of dementia is crucial for effective treatment and intervention, as well as for providing appropriate support to individuals and their families.

PREVALENCE AND IMPACT ON SOCIETY

Dementia is a widespread condition affecting millions of people globally. The prevalence of dementia increases with age, making it a significant concern in aging populations.

As of recent estimates, approximately 55 million people worldwide are living with dementia, and this number is expected to rise as the global population ages. The impact on society is profound, with dementia contributing to increased healthcare costs, caregiver burden, and challenges in providing adequate care and support.

The societal impact of dementia extends beyond healthcare costs to include emotional and financial strains on families and caregivers. Caring for someone with dementia can be demanding and stressful, often leading to caregiver burnout. Additionally, the need for long-term care facilities and specialized services increases with the growing prevalence of dementia, placing additional pressure on healthcare systems and resources.

Efforts to address the impact of dementia include promoting awareness, improving access to care, and supporting research for better treatments and prevention strategies. Public health initiatives and community programs play a crucial role in enhancing support for those affected by dementia and their families, aiming to reduce the burden and improve the quality of life for individuals living with this condition.

IMPORTANCE OF EARLY DIAGNOSIS AND INTERVENTION

Early diagnosis of dementia is critical for effective management and care. Identifying dementia in its early stages allows for timely intervention, which can help in managing symptoms, slowing progression, and improving overall quality of life. Early diagnosis enables individuals and their families to make informed decisions about treatment options, care planning, and lifestyle adjustments.

Interventions at an early stage may include medical treatments, cognitive therapies, and lifestyle changes aimed at managing symptoms and enhancing cognitive function. Additionally, early diagnosis provides an opportunity for individuals to engage in support services, such as counseling and educational programs, which can help them navigate the challenges of living with dementia.

Early intervention also plays a significant role in preparing for the future, as it allows individuals and families to plan for long-term care needs and make legal and financial arrangements. Proactive management of dementia can lead to better outcomes and a higher quality of life, underscoring the importance of recognizing and addressing cognitive changes as soon as they arise.

CHAPTER TWO
DEMENTIA AND ITS IMPACT
EFFECTS ON INDIVIDUALS AND FAMILIES

Dementia profoundly impacts both individuals and their families, altering daily life in significant ways. For those diagnosed, cognitive decline affects memory, decision-making, and the ability to perform routine tasks.

This can lead to frustration and confusion, as familiar activities become challenging and personal independence is compromised. The individual may struggle with disorientation, difficulty communicating, and changes in behavior, which can be distressing and disheartening.

Families are also deeply affected, experiencing a shift in their roles and responsibilities. Caregivers often face increased physical and emotional demands as they adjust to new caregiving duties, which can include managing medication, coordinating medical appointments, and providing assistance with personal care. The dynamic within the family may change as roles shift, with some members taking on more caregiving responsibilities while others may feel helpless or overwhelmed.

Moreover, the impact extends to family relationships, as stress and tension may arise from the constant caregiving demands. This stress can lead to strained relationships among family members, who might have differing opinions on care strategies or experience emotional exhaustion. The adjustment period can be challenging as families navigate their new reality, balancing caregiving with maintaining their own well-being and personal lives.

EMOTIONAL AND PSYCHOLOGICAL IMPACT

The emotional and psychological impact of dementia is significant, affecting both the individual with the diagnosis and their caregivers. For individuals, the gradual loss of cognitive functions can lead to feelings of grief, frustration, and depression.

They may struggle with the awareness of their declining abilities, experiencing a profound sense of loss as they cope with changes in their mental and emotional state. The recognition of their condition and the resulting confusion can contribute to emotional distress.

Caregivers, too, are vulnerable to emotional strain. The constant demands of caregiving can lead to burnout, anxiety, and depression. The emotional burden of watching a loved one's cognitive abilities deteriorate, combined with the stress of caregiving duties, can be overwhelming.

Caregivers may experience feelings of isolation, guilt, and sadness as they navigate the challenges of providing care and maintaining their mental health.

Addressing these emotional and psychological impacts requires support and intervention. Mental health professionals can offer counseling and therapy to help individuals and caregivers manage their emotions and develop coping strategies.

Support groups can provide a space for sharing experiences and gaining emotional support from others in similar situations, helping to alleviate feelings of isolation and distress.

FINANCIAL AND SOCIAL IMPLICATIONS

Dementia incurs substantial financial and social implications, affecting both the individual and their family. The costs associated with dementia care can be significant, including medical expenses for treatments, medications, and therapies.

Additionally, there may be costs for home modifications to enhance safety, or for hiring professional caregivers if family members are unable to provide full-time care.

Socially, dementia can impact an individual's ability to participate in activities and maintain social connections. As cognitive functions decline, individuals may withdraw from social interactions, leading to isolation and reduced engagement with their community. This social withdrawal can impact family dynamics and limit the individual's quality of life.

The financial burden of dementia can strain family resources, potentially leading to adjustments in lifestyle and spending. Families might need to make difficult financial decisions, such as reallocating funds for care or considering long-term care options. Navigating these financial and social implications requires careful planning and access to resources and support services to manage the financial impact and maintain social connections.

COPING WITH THE DIAGNOSIS

Coping with a dementia diagnosis involves a multifaceted approach to managing both the emotional and practical aspects of the condition. The initial shock of diagnosis can be overwhelming, and individuals and families need to seek accurate information about the condition.

Understanding the disease, its progression, and available treatments can help in planning and making informed care decisions.

Developing a comprehensive care plan is crucial. This plan should include medical treatment options, daily care routines, and legal and financial considerations. Engaging with healthcare professionals, such as neurologists and geriatricians, can guide managing symptoms and accessing appropriate resources. Additionally, involving a care team, including family members and professional caregivers, can help in managing the day-to-day challenges of dementia care.

Emotional support is equally important. Seeking counseling or joining support groups can provide valuable emotional relief and practical advice. Connecting with others who are experiencing similar challenges can offer comfort and insight into effective coping strategies. Building a support network and maintaining open communication with healthcare providers and loved ones can help individuals and families navigate the complexities of dementia.

SUPPORT SYSTEMS AND RESOURCES

Accessing support systems and resources is vital for managing dementia effectively. Various organizations and services offer assistance, ranging from educational resources to practical support. Alzheimer's associations and similar organizations provide valuable information on dementia, including resources for care planning, support groups, and caregiver training.

Professional caregiving services are available to assist with daily activities, providing respite for family caregivers. These services can include in-home care, adult day programs, and residential care options, depending on the level of care required. Evaluating these options can help families find the best fit for their needs and ensure that individuals with dementia receive appropriate care.

Community resources, such as local support groups and advocacy organizations, can offer additional assistance and a sense of community.

These groups provide emotional support, practical advice, and opportunities for social engagement. Utilizing these resources can help individuals and families manage the challenges of dementia more effectively and enhance their overall quality of life.

CHAPTER THREE

BASICS OF BRAIN FUNCTION AND AGING

HOW THE BRAIN FUNCTIONS NORMALLY

The human brain operates through an intricate network of neurons that transmit electrical signals. These neurons are organized into various regions, each responsible for different functions such as movement, sensation, and cognition. Neurotransmitters, which are chemical messengers, facilitate communication between neurons by crossing synapses, the small gaps between them.

This process allows the brain to process information, control bodily functions, and respond to external stimuli effectively.

In a well-functioning brain, these neural pathways are robust and capable of efficient communication. This efficiency supports learning, memory, and complex cognitive functions. The brain's plasticity, or its ability to adapt and reorganize itself by forming new connections, plays a crucial role in maintaining these functions throughout life. Regular mental and physical activities, such as problem-solving tasks and exercise, can enhance cognitive functions and support overall brain health.

Additionally, the brain is protected by several layers, including the blood-brain barrier, which prevents harmful substances from entering. This barrier ensures that the brain remains in a stable environment, supporting its normal function. Adequate nutrition, sleep, and stress management contribute to the optimal operation of the brain by providing essential nutrients and maintaining a balanced internal environment.

CHANGES IN THE BRAIN WITH AGING

As individuals age, the brain undergoes several structural and functional changes. One notable change is the gradual reduction in brain volume, particularly in the hippocampus and prefrontal cortex, areas crucial for memory and executive functions. This shrinkage can lead to slower cognitive processing and difficulties with memory retrieval. Additionally, the production of neurotransmitters may decrease, affecting communication between neurons and contributing to cognitive decline.

The aging brain also experiences a reduction in the number of neurons and synaptic connections. This decline can impair cognitive functions, such as learning and problem-solving, as the brain's ability to form new connections diminishes.

While some level of cognitive decline is normal with aging, significant changes can impact daily functioning and quality of life.

Despite these changes, the brain retains a degree of plasticity throughout life. Engaging in mental and physical exercises can help mitigate some of the cognitive decline associated with aging.

Activities such as puzzles, reading, and regular physical exercise can promote brain health and support cognitive functions by stimulating neural activity and maintaining neural connections.

HOW DEMENTIA AFFECTS BRAIN FUNCTION

Dementia is an umbrella term for a range of conditions characterized by a progressive decline in cognitive functions. Alzheimer's disease, the most common form of dementia, leads to the accumulation of amyloid plaques and tau tangles in the brain.

These abnormal structures disrupt neuronal communication, leading to the death of brain cells and significant cognitive impairment. As the disease progresses, affected individuals experience worsening memory loss, confusion, and difficulties with language and reasoning.

Other forms of dementia, such as vascular dementia, are caused by reduced blood flow to the brain, often due to stroke or other vascular conditions. This impaired blood flow results in damage to brain tissue, affecting cognitive functions.

Symptoms of vascular dementia may include problems with planning, judgment, and memory, which can vary depending on the specific areas of the brain affected.

Frontotemporal dementia affects the frontal and temporal lobes, leading to changes in personality, behavior, and language. Unlike Alzheimer's disease, which primarily affects memory, frontotemporal dementia causes significant changes in social behavior and executive functions. This form of dementia can make it challenging for individuals to manage everyday tasks and maintain social relationships.

EARLY SIGNS AND SYMPTOMS

Early signs of dementia often include subtle changes in memory, language, and behavior that are noticeable to close family and friends. Individuals may experience difficulty remembering recent events or conversations, struggling to find the right words during conversations, or becoming increasingly disoriented in familiar environments. These changes can start gradually and might be mistaken for normal age-related memory loss.

Behavioral changes, such as increased confusion or mood swings, can also be early indicators of dementia. Individuals may exhibit unusual behaviors, such as repetitive questioning, getting lost in familiar places, or displaying a lack of interest in previously enjoyed activities.

These symptoms can interfere with daily activities and relationships, making it important to monitor changes in behavior and cognition.

As dementia progresses, these early signs become more pronounced, affecting an individual's ability to perform routine tasks and maintain independence. Recognizing these symptoms early on is crucial for seeking appropriate medical advice and intervention, which can help manage the condition and improve the quality of life for those affected.

DIAGNOSIS AND ASSESSMENT

Diagnosing dementia involves a comprehensive assessment by healthcare professionals, including a detailed medical history, physical examination, and cognitive testing. Initial assessments may include a series of tests to evaluate memory, problem-solving abilities, and other cognitive functions. These tests help determine the extent of cognitive impairment and identify patterns consistent with various types of dementia.

Neuroimaging techniques, such as MRI or CT scans, are often used to visualize structural changes in the brain. These images can reveal atrophy in specific brain regions, such as the hippocampus in Alzheimer's disease, or identify vascular abnormalities in cases of vascular dementia. Blood tests may also be conducted to rule out other conditions that could cause similar symptoms.

In some cases, a neuropsychological evaluation may be performed to assess cognitive functions more thoroughly and differentiate between dementia and other potential causes of cognitive decline. This comprehensive approach allows for a more accurate diagnosis and helps tailor treatment and management strategies to the specific needs of the individual.

CHAPTER FOUR

TYPES OF DEMENTIA

ALZHEIMER'S DISEASE

Alzheimer's disease is the most common form of dementia, characterized by progressive memory loss and cognitive decline. This neurodegenerative condition is marked by the buildup of amyloid plaques and tau tangles in the brain, which disrupt communication between neurons and lead to cell death.

Symptoms typically begin with mild memory lapses and can advance to severe cognitive impairment, affecting daily living activities and personal independence.

Diagnosis involves a comprehensive assessment including medical history, cognitive testing, and brain imaging to rule out other causes of dementia. Treatment focuses on managing symptoms with medications such as cholinesterase inhibitors, which may help to improve or stabilize symptoms temporarily. Non-pharmacological interventions, such as cognitive therapies and support groups, also play a crucial role in enhancing quality of life.

Care for individuals with Alzheimer's requires a multidisciplinary approach. This includes personalized care plans, support for caregivers, and strategies to address behavioral symptoms. Engaging patients in structured routines and cognitive stimulation activities can help maintain cognitive function and slow the progression of symptoms while creating a supportive environment that ensures their safety and well-being.

VASCULAR DEMENTIA

Vascular dementia arises from reduced blood flow to the brain, often due to stroke or small vessel disease, which impairs brain function. The condition can present with sudden changes following a stroke or gradually worsening cognitive abilities, including difficulties with planning, organization, and memory.

The severity and progression depend on the location and extent of the brain damage.

Diagnosis of vascular dementia involves assessing vascular risk factors, such as hypertension and diabetes, alongside brain imaging techniques like MRI or CT scans. Treatment aims to manage underlying conditions that contribute to vascular damage, such as controlling blood pressure and cholesterol levels. Medications may be used to improve cognitive symptoms and prevent further vascular incidents.

Management of vascular dementia involves lifestyle modifications to improve cardiovascular health, such as adopting a healthy diet and regular physical activity. Cognitive therapies and rehabilitation can help individuals adapt to changes and maintain their independence. Coordination with healthcare providers to monitor and adjust treatment plans is essential for effective management.

LEWY BODY DEMENTIA

Lewy body dementia is characterized by the presence of Lewy bodies, which are abnormal protein deposits found in the brain that disrupt normal functioning. Symptoms include fluctuating cognitive abilities, visual hallucinations, and motor symptoms similar to Parkinson's disease, such as tremors and stiffness. Sleep disturbances and autonomic dysfunction may also occur, impacting daily life and well-being.

Diagnosing Lewy body dementia involves a thorough evaluation of symptoms, including cognitive tests, neuroimaging, and sometimes a brain biopsy to confirm the presence of Lewy bodies.

Treatment focuses on managing symptoms with medications like cholinesterase inhibitors for cognitive symptoms and Parkinson's disease medications for motor symptoms. Careful management is required as some medications used in other types of dementia can worsen symptoms in Lewy body dementia.

Care strategies for Lewy body dementia include tailored approaches to address cognitive, motor, and psychiatric symptoms. Supportive therapies, such as physical and occupational therapy, can improve mobility and daily functioning. Creating a stable and predictable environment, along with addressing sleep and behavioral issues, helps in enhancing the quality of life for individuals with this condition.

FRONTOTEMPORAL DEMENTIA

Frontotemporal dementia (FTD) involves degeneration of the frontal and temporal lobes of the brain, leading to changes in personality, behavior, and language. This type of dementia often presents with pronounced personality changes, social inappropriateness, and difficulty with language and communication. Unlike Alzheimer's disease, memory loss is not the primary early symptom.

Diagnosis of FTD requires a detailed clinical assessment, including neurological exams and imaging studies to differentiate it from other dementias. Genetic testing may be considered if there is a family history of the disease. While there are no specific treatments for FTD, management focuses on symptomatic relief and supportive care, including behavioral therapies and medications to address specific symptoms.

Care for individuals with FTD involves strategies to manage behavioral changes and support communication difficulties. Providing structured environments and clear routines can help reduce confusion and agitation. Engaging with support services for caregivers and families is crucial in navigating the challenges associated with this progressive condition.

OTHER LESS COMMON TYPES

Other less common types of dementia include conditions like Creutzfeldt-Jakob disease, which is characterized by rapid cognitive decline and motor symptoms due to prion infection, and normal pressure hydrocephalus, which involves fluid accumulation in the brain ventricles leading to walking difficulties and cognitive issues. Each type has distinct features and progression patterns, making accurate diagnosis essential.

Diagnosis typically involves a combination of clinical evaluation, brain imaging, and sometimes lumbar puncture to assess fluid dynamics or prion presence. Treatment varies depending on the type and may include medications to manage symptoms or surgical interventions in cases like normal pressure hydrocephalus. Early and precise diagnosis is critical for optimizing treatment and management.

Management strategies for these less common dementias often include specialized care plans and supportive therapies tailored to the specific symptoms and needs of the individual. Coordinating care with a multidisciplinary team ensures comprehensive support and adaptation to the unique challenges presented by these rarer forms of dementia.

CHAPTER FIVE

RISK FACTORS AND PREVENTION

GENETIC AND ENVIRONMENTAL RISK FACTORS

Genetic factors play a significant role in the risk of developing dementia. Individuals with a family history of dementia, particularly Alzheimer's disease, are at higher risk due to inherited genetic mutations. Certain genes, such as APOE4, have been linked to an increased likelihood of dementia. Understanding your family medical history can help you gauge your risk level and inform preventive measures. Genetic testing might be an option for those with a strong family history, although it's essential to discuss potential implications with a healthcare professional.

Environmental factors also contribute to dementia risk. Exposure to toxins, pollutants, and even lifestyle choices such as smoking can influence brain health. Additionally, conditions like chronic stress and social isolation have been linked to an increased risk of cognitive decline. Addressing these environmental factors involves making lifestyle changes and adopting healthier habits to mitigate their impact on brain health.

Mitigating genetic and environmental risks involves proactive strategies. Regular mental and physical health screenings can help detect early signs of cognitive decline. Implementing a healthy lifestyle, such as reducing exposure to pollutants and maintaining a supportive social network, can also contribute to lowering the risk. By being aware of these risk factors and taking preventive actions, individuals can better manage their overall risk of developing dementia.

LIFESTYLE FACTORS AND PREVENTION STRATEGIES

Lifestyle choices significantly impact dementia risk and overall brain health. Engaging in regular physical activity is crucial, as exercise improves blood flow to the brain and supports cognitive function.

Incorporating activities like walking, swimming, or cycling into your routine can enhance cardiovascular health and reduce dementia risk. Aim for at least 150 minutes of moderate exercise per week to maintain optimal brain health.

Mental stimulation and social engagement are also key factors in dementia prevention. Activities that challenge the brain, such as puzzles, reading, or learning new skills, can help maintain cognitive function. Additionally, staying socially active by participating in group activities, volunteering, or maintaining strong social connections can provide mental stimulation and emotional support, reducing the risk of cognitive decline.

Preventive strategies also include avoiding harmful habits and adopting healthy behaviors. Smoking cessation, moderate alcohol consumption, and managing chronic conditions like hypertension and diabetes can reduce dementia risk.

ROLE OF DIET AND EXERCISE

Diet plays a crucial role in maintaining brain health and reducing the risk of dementia. A balanced diet rich in antioxidants, omega-3 fatty acids, and essential vitamins supports cognitive function. Foods such as berries, leafy greens, fatty fish, and nuts are beneficial for brain health. The Mediterranean diet, which emphasizes fruits, vegetables, whole grains, and healthy fats, has been associated with a reduced risk of cognitive decline.

Exercise complements a healthy diet by improving blood circulation and enhancing brain function. Engaging in physical activities like aerobic exercises, strength training, and flexibility exercises can support overall cognitive health. Regular exercise not only helps with weight management but also reduces inflammation and oxidative stress, factors that contribute to dementia.

Combining a nutritious diet with regular exercise creates a comprehensive approach to brain health.

Maintaining this dual focus can help prevent cognitive decline and support long-term brain function.

COGNITIVE TRAINING AND MENTAL STIMULATION

Cognitive training and mental stimulation are essential for preserving cognitive function and reducing dementia risk. Engaging in brain-training exercises, such as memory games, problem-solving tasks, and cognitive puzzles, can enhance mental agility and support cognitive health. These activities challenge the brain and help build cognitive reserves, potentially delaying the onset of dementia.

Incorporating diverse mental stimulation activities into daily life is beneficial. Learning new skills, such as playing a musical instrument or speaking a new language, can provide significant cognitive benefits. Additionally, social interactions and discussions with others can stimulate the brain and promote mental health, reducing the risk of cognitive decline.

Adopting a routine that includes regular cognitive and social activities helps maintain mental sharpness.

IMPORTANCE OF REGULAR MEDICAL CHECK-UPS

Regular medical check-ups are vital for monitoring brain health and detecting early signs of dementia. Routine evaluations by a healthcare professional can help identify risk factors and provide personalized recommendations for maintaining cognitive health. These check-ups may include cognitive assessments, screenings for cardiovascular health, and evaluations of overall well-being.

Early detection through medical check-ups enables timely intervention and management of potential risk factors. Addressing issues such as hypertension, diabetes, or cholesterol levels can help reduce the risk of cognitive decline. Regular monitoring allows for adjustments to lifestyle and treatment plans based on individual health needs.

CHAPTER SIX
DIAGNOSIS AND TREATMENT
DIAGNOSTIC PROCESS AND TOOLS

Diagnosing dementia involves a comprehensive assessment to determine if a person has the condition and, if so, what type. The process typically begins with a detailed medical history and a review of symptoms. Doctors use various tools, such as the Mini-Mental State Examination (MMSE) or the Montreal Cognitive Assessment (MoCA), to evaluate cognitive functions including memory, attention, and problem-solving skills. These standardized tests help identify patterns of cognitive decline consistent with dementia.

Imaging studies like magnetic resonance imaging (MRI) or computed tomography (CT) scans are employed to visualize structural changes in the brain, such as atrophy or abnormalities that may indicate dementia.

Additionally, positron emission tomography (PET) scans can be used to assess brain activity and detect amyloid plaques, which are associated with Alzheimer's disease. Blood tests may also be conducted to rule out other potential causes of cognitive impairment, such as vitamin deficiencies or thyroid disorders.

Collaboration between specialists often aids in accurate diagnosis. Neurologists, geriatricians, and psychiatrists may work together to interpret results from cognitive tests and imaging studies.

A thorough assessment ensures that the diagnosis is accurate and helps guide the selection of appropriate treatment strategies tailored to the individual's specific needs.

MEDICAL AND COGNITIVE ASSESSMENTS

Medical assessments for dementia focus on evaluating both physical and cognitive health. Initially, a healthcare provider performs a comprehensive physical examination to identify any underlying health issues that might impact cognitive function. This includes reviewing the patient's medical history, current medications, and any recent changes in health status. Cognitive assessments, on the other hand, are designed to measure different aspects of mental function, including memory, reasoning, and language skills.

Cognitive tests often involve structured questions and tasks to evaluate memory recall, problem-solving abilities, and attention. For example, patients may be asked to remember a list of words or solve simple mathematical problems.

The results from these assessments provide valuable information about the severity and nature of cognitive decline, helping to differentiate between various types of dementia and other potential causes of cognitive issues.

In addition to these assessments, behavioral and psychological evaluations may be conducted to understand the impact of cognitive decline on daily living and emotional well-being. This holistic approach ensures that all aspects of the individual's health are considered in the diagnosis, leading to a more accurate understanding of their condition and the development of a tailored care plan.

AVAILABLE TREATMENTS AND MEDICATIONS

Treatment for dementia aims to manage symptoms and improve quality of life, rather than cure the condition. Medications such as cholinesterase inhibitors—donepezil, rivastigmine, and galantamine—are commonly prescribed to help with cognitive symptoms by increasing levels of neurotransmitters involved in memory and learning. Memantine, another medication, is used to regulate the activity of glutamate, a neurotransmitter that plays a role in memory and learning, helping to manage more severe symptoms.

Non-pharmacological treatments, including cognitive therapies and lifestyle changes, also play a crucial role in managing dementia. Cognitive stimulation therapy (CST) involves structured activities and exercises that help improve cognitive function and maintain mental abilities. Occupational therapy can assist individuals in adapting their environment and daily routines to better manage their symptoms and maintain independence.

It is important to monitor the effectiveness of treatments regularly and adjust them as needed. Healthcare providers work closely with patients and their families to evaluate the impact of medications and therapies, ensuring that any side effects are managed and that the treatment plan remains aligned with the individual's evolving needs.

ROLE OF CAREGIVERS AND FAMILY SUPPORT

Caregivers and family members are integral to the management and support of individuals with dementia. They provide essential daily care, including assistance with personal hygiene, medication management, and transportation to medical appointments. Caregivers often act as advocates for the patient, communicating their needs and preferences to healthcare providers and ensuring they receive appropriate care and support.

Emotional support is also a critical aspect of caregiving. Individuals with dementia may experience confusion, frustration, and emotional distress, and having a compassionate caregiver can help alleviate some of these challenges. Family members are encouraged to offer reassurance, engage in meaningful activities, and maintain open lines of communication to help improve the individual's overall well-being.

Support groups and counseling services can provide caregivers with additional resources and emotional support. These groups offer a space to share experiences, gain insights from others in similar situations, and learn about effective caregiving strategies. By connecting with these resources, caregivers can better manage the demands of their role and maintain their health and resilience.

ONGOING RESEARCH AND ADVANCEMENTS

Ongoing research into dementia aims to enhance understanding, improve diagnostic methods, and develop new treatments. Researchers are investigating the underlying causes of dementia, such as genetic factors and brain pathology, to uncover potential targets for therapeutic interventions. Studies on biomarkers and imaging techniques are exploring ways to identify dementia at earlier stages, which could lead to more effective treatments.

Clinical trials are testing new medications and therapies to address various aspects of dementia, including memory loss, behavioral symptoms, and disease progression. Advances in precision medicine and personalized approaches are offering hope for treatments tailored to the individual's specific type of dementia and genetic profile, potentially improving outcomes and reducing side effects.

In addition to drug development, research is focusing on non-pharmacological approaches such as cognitive rehabilitation, lifestyle interventions, and technology-assisted therapies. These advancements aim to provide comprehensive care strategies that enhance the quality of life for individuals with dementia and their families. As research progresses, new findings and innovations continue to shape the future of dementia care and management.

CHAPTER SEVEN

MANAGING DEMENTIA SYMPTOMS

BEHAVIORAL AND PSYCHOLOGICAL SYMPTOMS

Dementia can manifest through a range of behavioral and psychological symptoms, which often include agitation, aggression, delusions, and mood swings. These symptoms can be distressing for both individuals and their caregivers.

Agitation might present as restlessness or an inability to sit still, while aggression can include physical or verbal outbursts. Delusions may involve false beliefs, such as thinking that someone is stealing from them, while mood swings can lead to rapid changes in emotional states. Recognizing these symptoms is the first step in managing them effectively.

Managing these symptoms involves understanding the underlying causes and triggers. For instance, agitation might be linked to unmet needs such as hunger or discomfort, while aggression could stem from frustration or confusion. By identifying these triggers, caregivers can address them proactively. It is also important to communicate calmly and clearly with individuals showing these symptoms to avoid escalating the situation further. Utilizing comfort measures like familiar objects or music can also help soothe agitation and mood swings.

Caregivers should document changes in behavior to identify patterns and potential triggers. This information can be invaluable when consulting with healthcare professionals.

Regular updates can aid in adjusting treatment plans and interventions, ensuring that the approach remains effective as symptoms evolve. Collaboration with medical professionals, such as geriatricians or neurologists, can provide additional strategies tailored to the individual's specific needs.

TECHNIQUES FOR MANAGING CHALLENGING BEHAVIORS

Managing challenging behaviors in dementia involves employing various techniques to de-escalate and address these issues effectively. One effective technique is to use distraction and redirection to shift the individual's focus from a challenging behavior to a more positive or neutral activity.

For example, if an individual is agitated about a specific issue, redirecting their attention to a favorite activity or hobby can help reduce agitation and improve mood.

Another approach involves modifying the environment to reduce triggers that might lead to challenging behaviors. This could mean minimizing clutter, reducing noise levels, or creating a calm and soothing space. Ensuring that the environment is structured and predictable can help individuals with dementia feel more secure and less likely to act out. Simplifying tasks and providing clear, concise instructions can also prevent frustration and subsequent behavioral issues.

It's also important for caregivers to remain patient and maintain a calm demeanor when dealing with challenging behaviors.

Emotional reactions from caregivers can sometimes exacerbate the situation. Implementing structured routines and engaging in activities that the individual enjoys can further help in reducing the frequency and intensity of challenging behaviors.

STRATEGIES FOR IMPROVING QUALITY OF LIFE

Improving the quality of life for individuals with dementia involves a multi-faceted approach focused on enhancing daily living experiences. Creating a supportive and stimulating environment is crucial. This can include incorporating familiar items and routines, which can provide comfort and a sense of normalcy. Engaging in activities that match the individual's interests and abilities, such as art or music therapy, can also significantly enhance their overall well-being.

Social interactions and maintaining connections with loved ones play a vital role in improving quality of life. Encouraging regular social activities and fostering relationships can prevent feelings of isolation and loneliness. Structured social activities, whether within a group setting or through one-on-one interactions, help maintain cognitive function and emotional health.

Personalized care plans that address individual preferences and needs are essential. Regular assessments by healthcare professionals can help tailor these plans to better suit the evolving needs of the person with dementia.

This personalized approach ensures that care remains effective and responsive, contributing to an improved quality of life.

IMPORTANCE OF ROUTINE AND STRUCTURE

Routine and structure provide a sense of stability and predictability for individuals with dementia, which can greatly aid in managing their symptoms. Establishing consistent daily routines helps reduce confusion and anxiety, as individuals know what to expect and when. For instance, having regular meal times, bedtime routines, and scheduled activities can create a comforting and predictable environment.

Structured environments also contribute to safety and independence. For example, organizing the living space in a way that minimizes hazards and provides clear, easily navigable pathways can prevent accidents and confusion. Using visual cues, such as labels and signs, can assist individuals in recognizing where items are and what activities are next, further supporting their independence.

Incorporating routine into daily life also helps manage behavioral symptoms by providing a sense of normalcy.

Consistent routines can help alleviate agitation and reduce the frequency of challenging behaviors by creating a structured and secure environment. Caregivers should aim to create and maintain these routines, adapting them as necessary based on the individual's needs and abilities.

ROLE OF OCCUPATIONAL THERAPY AND SUPPORT SERVICES

Occupational therapy plays a crucial role in supporting individuals with dementia by helping them maintain independence and enhance their daily functioning. Occupational therapists assess the individual's abilities and create customized interventions that focus on improving skills necessary for daily living. This might include training in techniques for managing personal care, household tasks, or adapting activities to better suit their capabilities.

Support services, such as adult day care centers and respite care, provide additional assistance by offering structured activities and social interaction opportunities. These services can also give caregivers much-needed breaks, reducing their stress and preventing burnout. Access to community resources and support groups can offer practical advice, emotional support, and respite care options, contributing to a more balanced caregiving experience.

Coordination with healthcare professionals ensures that the individual's needs are continuously assessed and addressed. Regular consultations with medical providers, including geriatricians and neurologists, can help adapt treatment plans and interventions. Integrating occupational therapy with other support services provides a comprehensive approach to managing dementia, improving the overall quality of care and life for both individuals and their caregivers.

CHAPTER EIGHT

CAREGIVING AND SUPPORT

RESPONSIBILITIES OF CAREGIVERS

Caregivers for individuals with dementia face a range of responsibilities that require both physical and emotional stamina. Their primary duty is to provide daily assistance with activities of daily living (ADLs), which include bathing, dressing, and feeding. This assistance extends to managing medication schedules, monitoring changes in health, and ensuring safety within the home environment. Caregivers must also coordinate with healthcare professionals, manage appointments, and follow medical advice to maintain the person's health and well-being.

In addition to physical care, caregivers offer emotional support to individuals with dementia. This includes engaging them in meaningful activities, providing companionship, and helping them maintain a sense of normalcy and dignity.

Communication is vital, and caregivers must adapt their approach as the person's cognitive abilities decline. Effective communication helps in understanding their needs and reducing frustration or agitation.

Caregivers often handle household tasks and coordinate with other family members or professionals to ensure that all aspects of care are managed efficiently. This can involve organizing the home to be dementia-friendly, managing finances related to care, and addressing any behavioral challenges that may arise. Balancing these responsibilities requires careful planning and time management to provide comprehensive support while maintaining quality care.

BALANCING CAREGIVING WITH PERSONAL LIFE

Balancing caregiving with personal life is a challenging aspect of the caregiver's role. Caregivers must manage their health, relationships, and responsibilities while providing care. Establishing a routine that integrates caregiving tasks with personal time is crucial.

Creating a schedule that includes time for rest, social activities, and self-care helps prevent burnout and maintains overall well-being.

Setting boundaries is an essential part of this balance. Caregivers should communicate openly with family and friends about their needs and limitations. Involving other family members or seeking external help can alleviate some of the caregiving burdens and allow caregivers to focus on their personal lives. Prioritizing tasks and delegating responsibilities when possible helps in managing both caregiving and personal commitments.

Utilizing time management strategies and setting realistic goals can also help in balancing these aspects. Caregivers should make time for activities that rejuvenate them, whether it's a hobby, exercise, or socializing.

Regular breaks and personal time contribute to maintaining a healthy balance, ensuring that caregivers can continue to provide quality care without sacrificing their own needs and happiness.

RESPITE CARE AND SUPPORT NETWORKS

Respite care provides temporary relief for primary caregivers, allowing them to take a break from their caregiving duties. This care can be arranged through professional services, such as in-home respite care or short-term stays in assisted living facilities.

Respite care services offer trained personnel who can handle the caregiving tasks, giving the primary caregiver time to rest or attend to other responsibilities.

Support networks are crucial for caregivers, offering emotional and practical support. Connecting with local or online support groups can provide a space to share experiences, gain advice, and receive encouragement from others in similar situations.

These networks often offer resources, educational opportunities, and social events that help caregivers feel less isolated and more empowered.

In addition to formal respite services, informal support from family, friends, and community organizations can also be valuable. Caregivers can seek assistance from loved ones for occasional help with caregiving tasks or emotional support. Building a network of supportive individuals and organizations helps in managing the challenges of caregiving and ensures that caregivers have access to the resources they need.

LEGAL AND FINANCIAL CONSIDERATIONS

Legal and financial planning is essential for managing dementia care effectively. Caregivers should understand and arrange for legal documents such as power of attorney and advance directives, which allow for decisions to be made on behalf of the person with dementia when they are no longer able to make them independently.

Consulting with an attorney who specializes in elder law can ensure that all legal aspects are addressed appropriately.

Financial management involves budgeting for caregiving expenses, including medical costs, home modifications, and professional care services. Caregivers should explore options such as government benefits, insurance, and financial assistance programs to help cover these costs. Keeping detailed records of expenses and financial planning can help in managing the financial aspects of care efficiently.

Estate planning is another critical area, involving the management of assets and the distribution of the estate. This may include setting up trusts, managing investments, and addressing inheritance issues. Working with a financial advisor can help in creating a comprehensive plan that addresses both current and future financial needs, ensuring that the financial aspects of caregiving are handled effectively.

TRAINING AND RESOURCES FOR CAREGIVERS

Training and resources are vital for caregivers to provide effective care and manage their responsibilities. Caregivers should seek training on dementia care techniques, including understanding the progression of the disease, managing behavioral symptoms, and using effective communication strategies. Workshops, online courses, and caregiver training programs can provide valuable knowledge and skills.

Accessing resources such as educational materials, support groups, and community services can enhance a caregiver's ability to manage care. Many organizations offer resources that cover various aspects of caregiving, from handling daily tasks to understanding legal and financial issues. Utilizing these resources can provide practical guidance and emotional support.

Continuous learning and staying updated on best practices in dementia care are essential.

Caregivers should take advantage of ongoing educational opportunities and remain informed about new treatments, caregiving techniques, and support services. By investing in training and resources, caregivers can improve their skills and provide better care while managing their well-being.

CHAPTER NINE

LEGAL AND ETHICAL CONSIDERATIONS

LEGAL RIGHTS OF INDIVIDUALS WITH DEMENTIA

Individuals with dementia retain legal rights under the law, though these rights may be impacted by their cognitive decline. It is crucial to understand that while dementia may affect their ability to make decisions, their rights to privacy, dignity, and fair treatment must still be upheld.

Legal protections exist to ensure that individuals with dementia are not discriminated against and that their rights to access healthcare, participate in decisions about their care, and engage in legal and financial transactions are respected as much as possible.

To safeguard these rights, legal representatives or caregivers may need to become involved. They can help ensure that any decisions made on behalf of the individual are in their best interest and are made concerning their wishes and preferences.

It is essential for caregivers and family members to be aware of the individual's rights and to act by legal and ethical standards, consulting with legal professionals when necessary to navigate any complex issues that may arise.

Monitoring and advocacy play a significant role in protecting the legal rights of individuals with dementia. Regular reviews of care plans, legal documents, and treatment options can help ensure that the individual's rights are being upheld and that any necessary adjustments are made in response to changes in their condition or preferences.

ADVANCE DIRECTIVES AND POWER OF ATTORNEY

Advance directives and power of attorney are vital tools in managing the care and legal affairs of individuals with dementia. Advance directives are legal documents that allow individuals to outline their healthcare preferences in advance, ensuring that their wishes regarding medical treatment are followed even if they become unable to communicate them.

These directives typically include a living will and a durable power of attorney for healthcare, which appoints someone to make medical decisions on their behalf.

The power of attorney for finances is another crucial document, granting a trusted person the authority to handle financial matters and legal decisions if the individual becomes incapacitated.

Setting up these documents while the individual is still competent is essential to ensure their preferences are respected and to avoid potential conflicts or complications in the future.

Creating and updating advance directives and power of attorney documents requires careful consideration and legal guidance. It's important to discuss these decisions with the individual, family members, and legal advisors to ensure that all aspects of their care and financial management are addressed according to their wishes and legal requirements.

ETHICAL DILEMMAS IN DEMENTIA CARE

Dementia care often presents complex ethical dilemmas, especially concerning autonomy, consent, and quality of life. Caregivers and healthcare providers must balance the need for safety and appropriate care with respect for the individual's autonomy and personal preferences. Ethical issues may arise when deciding between honoring the individual's wishes and making decisions that may protect them from harm but limit their freedom.

Decisions about interventions, medication, and lifestyle choices require careful ethical consideration. For instance, determining whether to implement a more restrictive care approach to ensure safety might conflict with the individual's right to live as freely as possible. Caregivers must weigh these factors while considering the individual's overall well-being and preferences.

Ethical decision-making in dementia care also involves communication and collaboration with the individual's family and support network. Open discussions and consultations with ethical committees or advisors can provide guidance and help navigate these challenging situations, ensuring that decisions are made in the best interest of the person with dementia while respecting their dignity and rights.

GUARDIANSHIP AND DECISION-MAKING

Guardianship may be necessary when an individual with dementia is no longer able to make informed decisions about their care or finances. Guardianship involves a legal process where a court appoints a guardian to make decisions on behalf of the individual. This process ensures that someone is legally authorized to act in the individual's best interest, especially when they cannot do so themselves.

The process for establishing guardianship typically requires proving the individual's incapacity through medical evaluations and legal hearings.

It's important to select a guardian who understands the individual's preferences and needs, and who will act responsibly and ethically in managing their affairs. Guardianship can involve various responsibilities, including managing finances, making healthcare decisions, and ensuring the individual's overall well-being.

In some cases, less restrictive alternatives to full guardianship may be available, such as limited guardianship or the appointment of a representative payee for specific financial matters. These alternatives can provide a balance between protecting the individual's interests and allowing them to retain as much independence as possible.

PROTECTING PERSONAL AND FINANCIAL INTERESTS

Protecting the personal and financial interests of individuals with dementia involves implementing measures to safeguard their assets and ensure their well-being. This includes managing their finances responsibly, setting up legal safeguards such as trusts, and monitoring their care to prevent abuse or neglect. Financial planning tools, such as setting up a durable power of attorney, can help manage the individual's finances and protect their assets from exploitation.

Caregivers and family members should regularly review financial accounts and transactions to detect any unusual activity or potential fraud. In addition, safeguarding personal information and ensuring that the individual's personal care environment is secure are essential steps in protecting their interests. This may involve hiring reputable caregivers, conducting background checks, and ensuring that all legal documents and safeguards are up-to-date.

Legal and financial professionals can provide valuable assistance in creating strategies to protect personal and financial interests.

CHAPTER TEN

FAQS

WHAT ARE THE COMMON SYMPTOMS OF DEMENTIA?

Dementia presents with a range of symptoms that primarily affect cognitive functions. Early signs often include memory loss, where individuals struggle to recall recent events or conversations. As the condition progresses, confusion regarding time and place becomes more frequent, causing difficulties in recognizing familiar locations or understanding the current day. Language problems, such as finding the right words or following conversations, are also common, impacting the ability to communicate effectively.

Behavioral changes are another hallmark of dementia, with individuals displaying personality shifts and mood swings. They may become withdrawn, anxious, or irritable, and their ability to perform routine tasks can decline.

This may manifest as challenges in managing finances, handling household chores, or following a recipe. As symptoms worsen, daily living skills are further compromised, leading to issues with self-care and maintaining personal hygiene.

Additionally, individuals with dementia often experience difficulty with problem-solving and judgment. Once easy tasks, such as planning a trip or handling complex activities, become overwhelming. They may also struggle with spatial awareness, resulting in accidents or getting lost. Understanding these symptoms helps in recognizing the condition early and seeking appropriate care and support.

HOW IS DEMENTIA DIAGNOSED?

Diagnosing dementia involves a comprehensive assessment conducted by healthcare professionals. The process begins with a detailed medical history and evaluation of symptoms. This includes gathering information from the patient, family members, or caregivers about changes in cognitive abilities, daily functioning, and behavioral patterns. This information helps create a baseline for comparison and assists in ruling out other conditions that might mimic dementia symptoms.

Neurological examinations play a crucial role in diagnosis. These assessments test cognitive function, including memory, attention, language, and problem-solving skills. Imaging studies, such as MRI or CT scans, are often used to identify structural changes in the brain that are characteristic of dementia, such as atrophy or lesions. Blood tests and other laboratory evaluations are also conducted to exclude other potential causes of cognitive decline, such as vitamin deficiencies or thyroid disorders.

In some cases, more specialized tests may be required. Neuropsychological testing provides a detailed analysis of cognitive functions, helping to differentiate between various types of dementia. Additionally, a definitive diagnosis might involve ruling out reversible causes of dementia and confirming that the symptoms meet the criteria for specific types of dementia, such as Alzheimer's disease or vascular dementia.

WHAT TREATMENTS ARE AVAILABLE FOR DEMENTIA?

Treatment for dementia focuses on managing symptoms and improving quality of life, as there is currently no cure for the condition. Medications are commonly prescribed to address cognitive symptoms and behavioral issues. Cholinesterase inhibitors, such as donepezil and rivastigmine, are used to enhance memory and cognitive function by increasing levels of neurotransmitters in the brain. Another class of drugs, memantine, helps regulate glutamate activity, which is involved in learning and memory.

In addition to pharmacological treatments, non-drug therapies are essential in managing dementia. Cognitive stimulation therapy, which involves engaging in activities and exercises, can help improve cognitive function and delay decline. Occupational therapy focuses on enhancing daily living skills and adapting the environment to ensure safety and independence. Behavioral therapies and counseling provide support for managing mood changes and challenging behaviors.

Supportive care is crucial for both patients and caregivers. This includes creating a structured routine, ensuring a safe living environment, and facilitating social interactions to reduce isolation. Care plans often involve a multidisciplinary approach, incorporating input from doctors, nurses, social workers, and therapists to provide comprehensive care tailored to the individual's needs.

HOW CAN CAREGIVERS TAKE CARE OF THEMSELVES?

Caregivers play a vital role in supporting individuals with dementia but often face significant stress and challenges. Caregivers must prioritize their well-being to maintain their ability to provide effective care. This begins with recognizing the importance of self-care and making time for activities that promote physical and mental health. Regular exercise, balanced nutrition, and adequate rest are fundamental in managing stress and maintaining energy levels.

Setting boundaries and seeking support are essential for caregivers. This may involve delegating responsibilities, utilizing respite care services, or joining support groups where caregivers can share experiences and receive guidance. Professional counseling or therapy can also provide valuable support in managing the emotional and psychological aspects of caregiving, helping caregivers cope with feelings of frustration or burnout.

Additionally, caregivers should be mindful of their own needs and seek medical attention when necessary. Regular check-ups and monitoring of personal health can prevent burnout and ensure that caregivers remain physically and emotionally equipped to handle the demands of caregiving. Building a strong support network, both personal and professional, can offer practical assistance and emotional relief.

WHAT IS THE ROLE OF RESEARCH IN DEMENTIA CARE?

Research plays a critical role in advancing dementia care by driving the development of new treatments, improving diagnostic methods, and enhancing the quality of life for patients. Ongoing research efforts focus on understanding the underlying mechanisms of dementia, identifying biomarkers for early diagnosis, and discovering potential therapeutic targets. This research helps in developing drugs and interventions that can slow or modify the progression of the disease.

Clinical trials are a key component of research, testing new treatments and therapies to evaluate their safety and effectiveness. These trials provide valuable data that informs clinical practice and guides treatment options. Participation in clinical trials offers patients access to cutting-edge therapies and contributes to the broader knowledge base that benefits the entire dementia community.

In addition to medical research, studies exploring caregiving strategies, patient support, and quality-of-life enhancements are essential. Research into non-pharmacological interventions, such as cognitive therapies and lifestyle modifications, helps improve day-to-day care and support for individuals with dementia. By integrating research findings into practice, healthcare providers can offer more effective and evidence-based care for those affected by dementia.

www.ingramcontent.com/pod-product-compliance
Lightning Source LLC
Chambersburg PA
CBHW070204230526
45471CB00002B/810